I Vow...

Samarri,
I appreciate you
and your journey.
I pray this book
is a blessing.

Geneva
McPherson

This to Me

Introduction

Have you ever reflected back to what life could have been or should have been? Relationships that have come and gone. Jobs and stability as we know it has come and gone. Family life has changed in some way. Those thoughts that sometimes cripples us from learning, growing, and changing as life is changing around us.

Life is a journey full of unexpected twists and turns, ups and downs, highs and lows. Today, I Vow to be good to me. I Vow to be fair to me. I Vow to be free. I Vow to be ME. Say it with ME... I VOW THIS TO ME.

Young Vows

I Vow to love you.
I Vow to cherish you.
I Vow to honor you.
I Vow to respect you.
I Vow to protect you.
I Vow to never hurt you.
I Vow to be your best friend.
I Vow to be what you need.
I Vow me to you.
I Vow this to you.
I Vow...

Complicated Vows

I Vow to understand.
I Vow to listen.
I Vow to hear.
I Vow to be available.
I Vow to be present.
I Vow to still love you.
I Vow to still honor you.
I Vow to remain.
I Vow this to you.
I Vow...

"Still" Vows

I Vow to STILL listen.
I Vow to STILL learn.
I Vow to STILL love.
I Vow to STILL lean on you.
I Vow to STILL remain.
I Vow to STILL honor you.
I Vow to STILL protect you.
I Vow to STILL be present.
I Vow this to you.
I Vow...

"Still" Complicated Vows

I Vow to try to STILL understand.
I Vow to try to STILL listen.
I Vow to try to STILL protect you.
I Vow to try to STILL hear you.
I Vow to try to STILL honor you.
I Vow to try to STILL remain.
I Vow this to you... STILL.
I Vow...

Understanding Vows

I Vow to understand your misunderstanding.
I Vow to listen when you don't want to be heard.
I Vow to learn when you don't want to teach.
I Vow to love when you don't want to love.
I Vow to hold you when you don't want to be held.
I Vow to fall in love with you when you fall out of love.
I Vow to be the mirror even when you don't want to look.
I Vow to be the good in you.
I Vow to see the good in you.
I Vow THIS to YOU.
I Vow...

"Mirror" Vows

I Vow to love you.
I Vow to cherish you.
I Vow to honor you.
I Vow to respect you.
I Vow to protect you.
I Vow to never hurt you.
I Vow to be your best friend.
I Vow to be what you need.
I Vow me to you.
I Vow this to you.
I Vow...

Older Vows

I Vow to be patient with you.
I Vow to be protective over you.
I Vow to be gentle with you.
I Vow to be kind to you.
I Vow to be generous to you.
I Vow to be respectful toward you.
I Vow to BE you.
I Vow this to you.
I Vow...

End Vows

I Vow... to try.

Reflection

No matter what comes and goes in life, I am worthy and I am capable. I am confident and competent. I can and I will.

I can and I will live my best life for ME.

I Vow this to ME.

...

Made in the USA
Middletown, DE
01 March 2018